SERVET

UPDATE

CLINICAL CASES
IN SMALL ANIMAL
DERMATOLOGY

Sandra Díaz

SERVET

For this English edition:

Servet Update. Clinical cases in small animal dermatology

Plaza Antonio Beltrán Martínez nº 1, planta 8 - letra I
(Centro empresarial El Trovador)
50002 Zaragoza - Spain

First printing: January 2018

This book has been published originally in Spanish under the title:
Servet Update. Casos clínicos de dermatología en pequeños animales

ISBN Spanish edition: 978-84-16818-76-1

Translation:
Shannon Taylor Jiménez

ISBN: 978-84-17225-27-8
D.L.: Z 1887-2017

Design, layout and printing:
Servet editorial - Grupo Asís Biomedia, S.L.
www.grupoasis.com
info@grupoasis.com

Servet is the publishing house of Grupo Asís

Warning:

Veterinary science is constantly evolving, as are pharmacology and the other sciences. Inevitably, it is therefore the responsibility of the veterinary surgeon to determine and verify the dosage, the method of administration, the duration of treatment and any possible contraindications to the treatments given to each individual patient, based on his or her professional experience. Neither the publisher nor the author can be held liable for any damage or harm caused to people, animals or properties resulting from the correct or incorrect application of the information contained in this book.

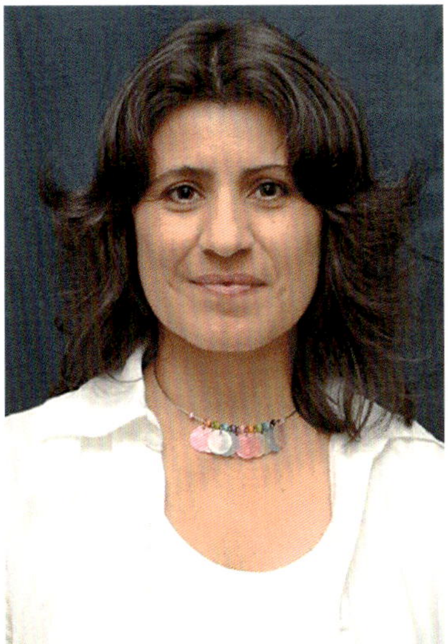

THE AUTHOR

Sandra Díaz

DVM, MS, Diplomate ACVD

Dr Sandra Díaz obtained her Doctor of Veterinary Medicine (DVM) degree from Santo Tomás University (Santiago, Chile) in 1996 and her Master of Science (MS) degree from the University of Minnesota (United States) in 2003, where she also completed her residency. She is board certified by the American College of Veterinary Dermatology (ACVD). Currently, she is an assistant professor in the Department of Dermatology and Otology at the College of Veterinary Medicine at Ohio State University (United States). She was previously assistant professor of dermatology in the Department of Small Animal Clinical Sciences at the Virginia-Maryland College of Veterinary Medicine (VMCVM) at Virginia Tech (United States). Before joining the faculty at the VMCVM, she was a member of the staff at the NYC Veterinary Specialists and Cancer Center, located in New York City. Her research interests focus on hair growth disorders, canine and feline allergic disorders and canine and feline otitis.

PREFACE

Canine and feline dermatitis and otitis are a frequent reason for consultation in veterinary medicine. Dermatitis can be caused by a number of agents, including external irritants, burns, allergens, traumas and infections (bacterial, viral, parasitic, or fungal). It can also be associated with concurrent internal or systemic illness, and hereditary factors may also be involved. Allergies form an important group of aetiological factors, especially in small animals.

The skin's response to an attack is known generally as dermatitis, which is expressed as any combination of pruritus, flaking, erythema, thickening, or lichenification of the skin, hyperpigmentation, seborrhoea oleosa, odor, and alopecia. The regular progression of a skin condition indicates an underlying problem that can cause primary lesions such as papules, pustules and blisters. Pruritus is a common clinical sign in many diseases, and in conditions that are not inherently pruritic, it can often occur due to secondary infections or as a result of inflammatory mediator production. As inflammatory changes progress, scabs and flakes form. If the process includes the deepest dermis, it can produce exudation, pain and fistulas or ulcers. Secondary bacterial and yeast infections commonly develop as a result of skin inflammation. As dermatitis becomes chronic, the acute signs of inflammation (such as erythema) disappear and primary lesions are obscured by signs of chronic inflammation (thickening of the skin, hyperpigmentation, flaking, seborrhoea). Often, the skin becomes drier. If pruritus is not a component of the primary disease, it will frequently develop at this stage. Successful treatment of dermatitis requires the identification of the underlying cause and treatment of secondary infections and other complications.

External otitis is the inflammation of the ear canal distal to the tympanic membrane, where the pinnae may or may not be involved. Otitis can be acute or chronic and unilateral or bilateral. Clinical signs can include agitation, odour, pain, exudate, and erythema. Causes of external otitis can be defined as primary or secondary, and there are also factors that can contribute, promote, or prevent the resolution of the condition. The best treatment for chronic otitis is prevention. The key to successful treatment is discussion with the owner about the known or suspected cause of the external otitis, if the otitis is curable, and if the underlying condition is going to require treatment for life, as is the case for atopic dermatitis. All the primary and secondary causes and risk factors should be identified and treated.

This book's objective is to show, from a practical point of view, how to manage dermatitis and otitis through case studies that include common conditions that represent diagnostic or management challenges, as well as less common diseases, such as the hepatocutaneous syndrome, in which identifying the cutaneous lesions helps us suspect the condition and come to a definitive diagnosis. Since the identification and distribution of the lesions are important to diagnose dermatological diseases, we hope that the images will aid the reader in recognising and learning about these skin diseases.

Sandra Díaz

TABLE OF CONTENTS

ATOPIC DERMATITIS

Canine atopic dermatitis (AD) is a pruritic disease with a complex aetiopathogenesis. By definition, AD is an inflammatory and pruritic skin disease with characteristic clinical signs. Affected individuals are genetically predisposed to develop IgE antibodies against environmental allergens. However, recent studies have demonstrated that AD is not always mediated by IgE. As also observed in humans, in a small subset of dogs with AD IgE is not detected by serological or intradermal testing. This form of AD has recently been named dermatitis similar to atopic dermatitis.

CLINICAL CASE. PEPE

Male American Pitbull Terrier, neutered, 4 years old.

PATIENT HISTORY

The patient had been suffering from severe pruritus for a year. On a scale of 1 to 10, with 1 being no pruritus and 10 being severe pruritus (see *Levels of pruritus in dogs*, page 8), the client rated the level of pruritus as an 8. The pruritus had worsened gradually over the previous 6 months, and was not stable but varied in intensity. Previous treatments included cephalexin via multiple 14-day treatments, and methylprednisolone acetate injections, which were normally administered monthly. Pepe had responded well, but the clinical signs had reappeared approximately one month after discontinuing the treatments. His diet was a chicken and rice–based, high-quality commercial diet.

CLINICAL EXAMINATION

Severe erythema was observed in the periocular area, rostral section of the nose, ventral neck, axillae (Fig. 1), inguinal area, ventral abdomen, interdigital areas (Fig. 2), and between the footpads. The nails had a reddish-brown discolouration and the nail area was eroded (Fig. 3). The skin of the ventral neck and axillae showed lichenification. Pustules and yellowish scabs were visible on the ventral abdomen (Fig. 4).

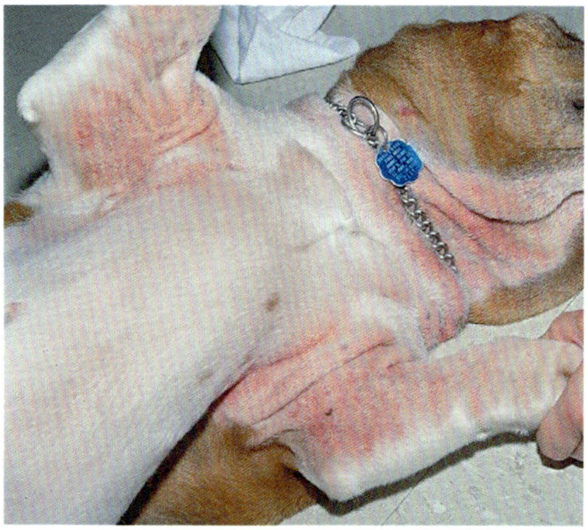

Figure 1. Severe erythema in the ventral area (neck, axillae, inner area of the upper limbs).

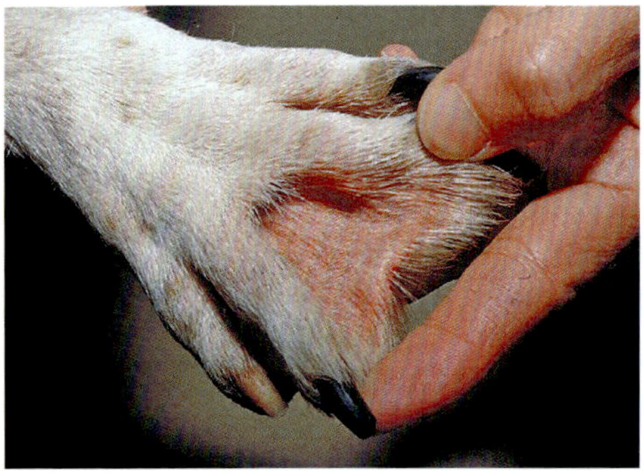

Figure 2. Severe erythema in the interdigital area.

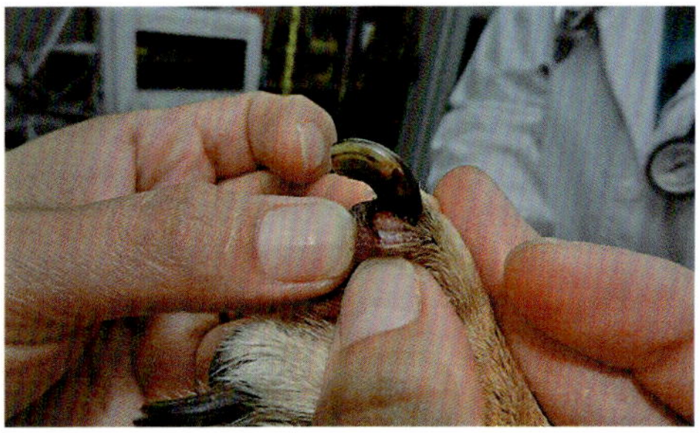

Figure 3. Reddish-brown discolouration on the nail and in the nail fold.

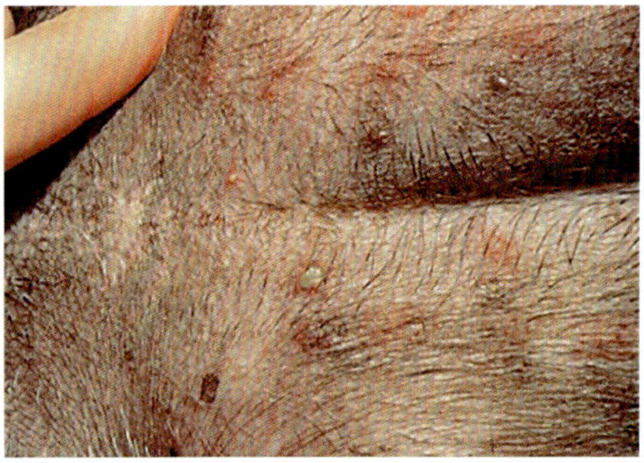

Figure 4. Yellowish pustules and scabs on the ventral abdomen.

Levels of pruritus in dogs

- **Extreme pruritus/almost constant**
  Scratches constantly, including when distracted, in all areas and at all times. Scratches during the appointment (physical restraint needed to keep the dog from scratching more).
- **Severe pruritus/prolonged episodes of pruritus**
  Wakes often to scratch or scratches while asleep. Also scratches while eating, playing, exercising, or while occupied with another activity.
- **Moderate pruritus/regular episodes**
  Wakes at night to scratch, but does not scratch while eating, playing, running, or while occupied with another activity.
- **Slight pruritus/more frequent than normal episodes**
  Does not scratch while sleeping, eating, playing, running, or when distracted by another activity.
- **Very slight pruritus/occasional episodes**
  Slight increase in itching when compared with when the dog did not have skin problems.
- **Normal dog**
  Does not scratch any more often than before the skin problems appeared.

DIFFERENTIAL DIAGNOSIS

Based on the history and clinical presentation. During the first visit, the following differential diagnoses were considered:

- AD: distribution of clinical signs, breed, age.
- Food allergy: distribution of clinical signs, breed, age.
- Demodicosis: severe erythema, pododermatitis, breed.
- Sarcoptic mange: though the distribution of the clinical signs was not characteristic, it was decided to include sarcoptic mange due to the level of pruritus.

The patient also presented with evidence of secondary problems:

- Superficial pyoderma.
- Paronychia.
- Pododermatitis.

DIAGNOSTIC TESTS

During this first visit, it was decided to perform:

- Surface scraping: to aid the diagnosis of sarcoptic mange.
- Deep scraping: to diagnose or rule out demodicosis.
- Skin cytology: to confirm the presence of secondary infections (*Staphylococcus, Malassezia*).

Skin scraping

- Choose an area that is normally affected, avoiding extremely traumatised areas. Perform the scraping with a spatula or a scalpel blade with mineral oil (Fig. 5):
  - *Demodex canis*: pinch the skin, release, and perform a deep scraping (until you observe capillary bleeding).
  - *Sarcoptes* spp.: perform surface scrapings.
- Transfer the material onto a slide with mineral oil and cover with a coverslip.
- Examine under 4× and 10× lenses. Lower the condenser to create more contrast.

Skin cytology

- The technique used varies according to the type and location of the lesion:
  - Impression smear (Fig. 6):
    - Surface of exudative lesions.
    - After opening a pustule.
    - After removing a scab.
  - Adhesive tape (transparent) (Fig. 7):
    - Oily or dry lesions.
    - Lesions that are difficult to reach with a slide.

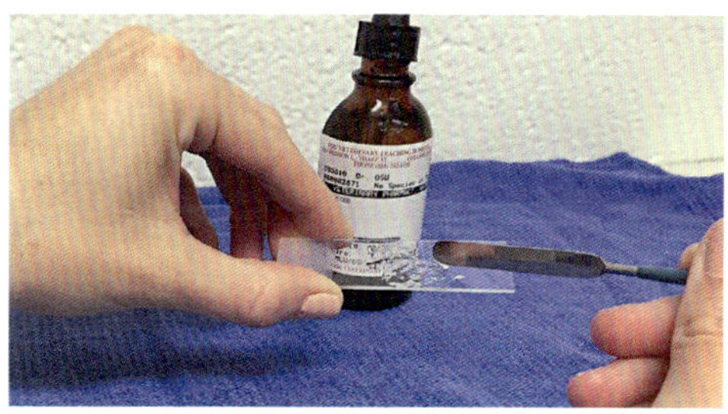

Figure 5. Materials used to perform skin scrapings: stainless steel spatula or No. 10 scalpel blade, mineral oil, slide, and coverslip.

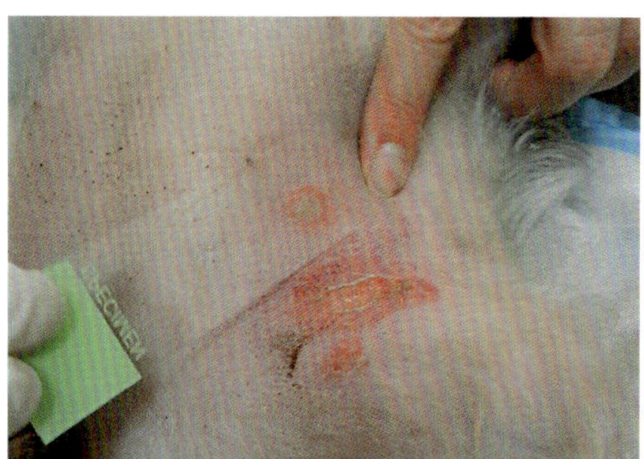

Figure 6. Impression smear of a pustule.

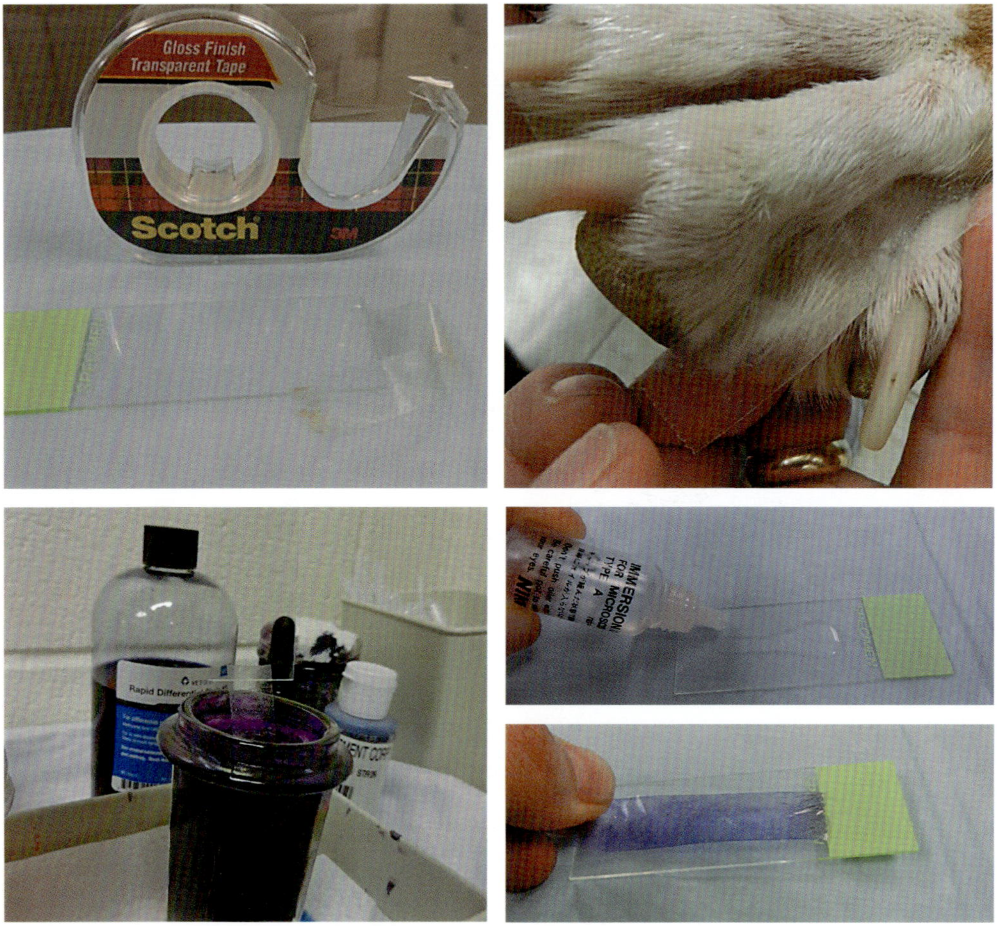

Figure 7. Adhesive tape applied in the interdigital area.

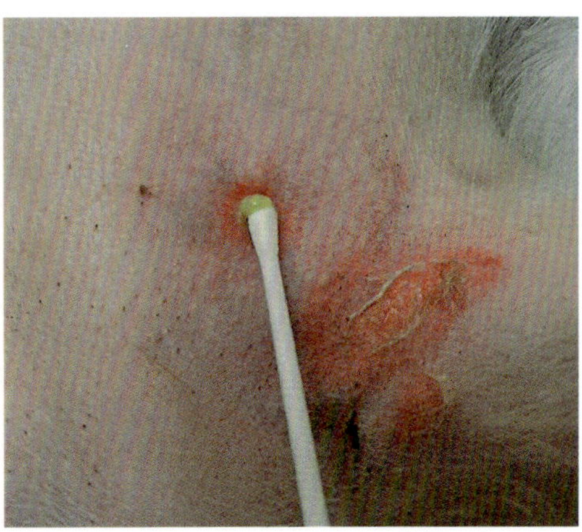

Figure 8. Swab of a pustule located in the inguinal area.

- Swab (Fig. 8):
    - Ears, exudative skin lesions.
- Spatula (if you do not have a stainless steel spatula you can use the wooden part of a swab) (Fig. 9):
    - Nail fold, paronychia.
- Dry the sample in the air or with a lighter and stain with Diff-Quik (air dry and use only the third reagent for adhesive tape).
- Examine the sample with a low magnification lens (4×).
- Identify areas of interest: e.g. inflammatory cells.
- Use immersion oil: 50–100× lens (adjust the condenser to a higher position).

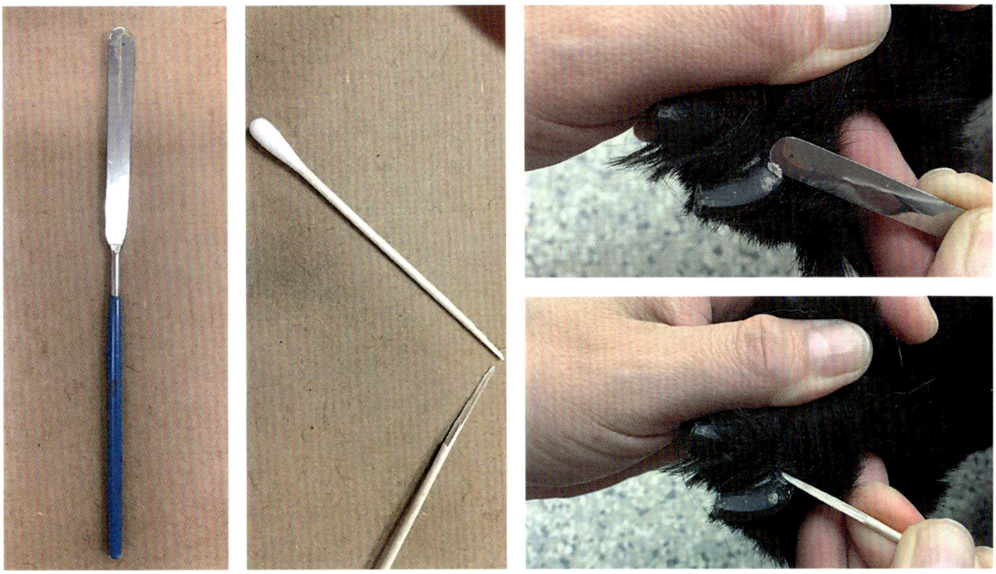

Figure 9. Taking samples from the nail area.

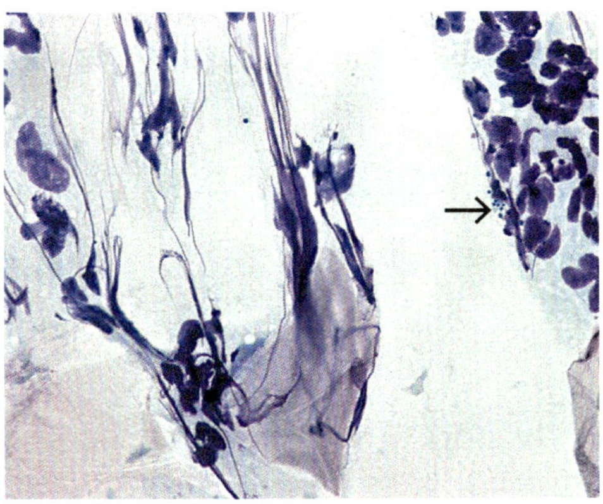

Figure 10. Presence of bacteria (arrow) in the impression smear from the inguinal area.

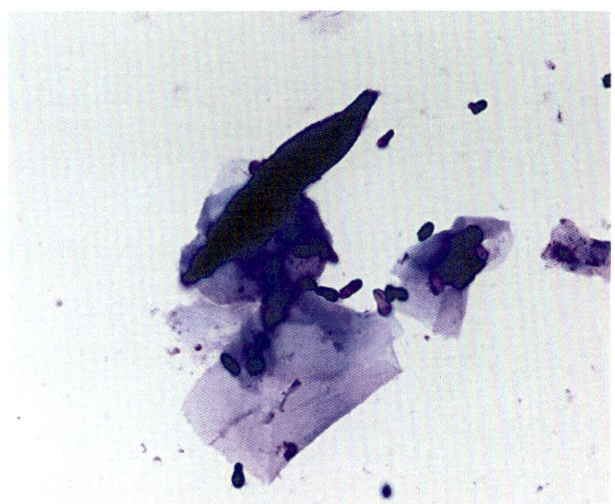

Figure 11. Presence of yeast in the interdigital area.

Results

The surface and deep scrapings were negative, so demodicosis was ruled out. It was decided to treat the patient for sarcoptic mange.

The cytological examination of the skin showed the presence of bacteria (Fig. 10) in the axillary area and ventral abdomen, as well as yeast in the nail folds and interdigital area (Fig. 11). Once the presence of bacteria was confirmed, a bacterial culture was performed since the patient had received several short-term cephalexin treatments.

TREATMENT

Based on the results of the diagnostic tests, it was decided to topically treat the pododermatitis, the paronychia due to yeast and the superficial pyoderma while waiting for the culture results.

The treatment included:

- Bathing with a chlorhexidine and miconazole shampoo twice a week, with a contact period of 5 to 10 minutes.
- Medicated wipes: between baths it was recommended to use acetic and boric acid wipes on the affected areas (neck, axillae, ventral abdomen, paws).
- Oclacitinib at 0.5 mg/kg every 24 hours for the control of pruritus.
- The culture showed the presence of *Staphylococcus pseudintermedius* sensitive to cephalosporins, so treatment was initiated with cephalexin at 30 mg/kg every 12 hours until the next visit.

A follow-up visit at 4 weeks was recommended.

Second visit

During the second visit, the client reported significant improvement and rated the level of pruritus as a 1–2 out of 10. No lesions were observed in the physical examination. Samples were taken from the nail folds and interdigital area to confirm the resolution of the yeast infection. The samples were negative.

Elimination diet

An elimination diet was recommended. The owner was instructed to feed the selected diet exclusively for 8–10 weeks and to avoid giving Pepe biscuits, bones, flavoured medications or medications in gel capsules, flavoured toothpaste, etc.

The client was given the option of a homemade or commercial diet, and the advantages and disadvantages of each were discussed.

Homemade diet

- Advantages:
  - Does not contain additives.
  - Only one source of protein.
- Disadvantages:
  - Not balanced.
  - Takes longer to prepare.

Commercial diet

- Advantages:
  - Easy.
  - Balanced.
- Disadvantages:
  - Usually uses more than one source of protein.
  - Contains additives.

Hydrolyzed commercial diet

Does not contain intact proteins, only peptides sized between 1,000 to 15,000 daltons.

It was decided to use a diet with limited ingredients based on kangaroo meat and oats.

Client education

The owner was asked to keep a diary to note:

- All food that was given to the dog or that the dog ate.
- Pruritus level.
- Stool characteristics.

Follow-up

- Follow-up visit 4 to 8 weeks later.
- What was expected?
  - 50 % show a response at 4 weeks.
  - If there was still no response, the diet would be continued for 4 more weeks.
- To evaluate the patient's response, oclacitinib was discontinued during the eighth week of implementation of the elimination diet. The patient showed a gradual increase in the level of pruritus over the course of the first week, and during the following visit (9 weeks after beginning the diet), the owner rated the level of pruritus as a 7 out of 10.
- It was determined that the most likely reason was an environmental allergy and the client was offered serological tests to identify the specific IgE allergen and an intradermal test. The advantages and disadvantages of both tests were explained to the client, and it was emphasised that these tests were performed primarily to select the allergens that would be included in an immunotherapy vaccine, since avoiding or reducing exposure to the allergens is difficult to implement.

Allergy tests

Intradermal test

Detects the presence of specific IgE antibodies adhered to mast cells in the dermis and tests the capacity of mast cells to release inflammatory mediators after exposure to specific allergens.

- Advantages:
  - Performed on the organ that is affected by the disease.
  - Fewer false positives when compared with serology.
  - Fast: the animal can begin immunotherapy as soon as the results are interpreted.
- Disadvantages:
  - Results can be affected by some medications.
  - Need to purchase the allergens.
  - Training is needed to perform the test and interpret it.
  - The dog must be sedated and its fur clipped.
  - Animals with AD can give negative results.

Allergen-specific IgE serology testing

Measures allergen-specific IgE present in the patient's serum.

- Advantages:
  - No need to sedate or clip the animal's fur.
  - Gives quantitative results.
  - Does not require training.
- Disadvantages:
  - Higher incidence of false positive reactions.
  - Low repeatability.

It was decided to perform both tests on the patient and combine the results to begin allergen-specific immunotherapy (Table 1). Oclacitinib treatment was reinitiated and the owner was informed that this medication would likely be necessary during the first 6–9 months of immunotherapy.

> Allergen-specific IgE serology is used to select the allergens to be employed in immunotherapy after a clinical diagnosis of atopic dermatitis.

Table 1. Results of the allergen-specific IgE serology tests. ≤10 (negative): allergen-specific IgE not detected; from 11 to 25 (+): allergen-specific IgE detected. In this category, the allergens should be considered for immunotherapy if exposure is consistent with the patient's history; from 26 to 50 (++): high levels of allergen-specific IgE detected. In this category, the allergens should be considered for immunotherapy if exposure is consistent with the patient's history; from 51 to >600 (+++): extremely high levels of allergen-specific IgE detected. In this category, the allergens should be considered first and foremost for immunotherapy if exposure is consistent with the patient's history.

		Results according to HERBU™
Grasses	*Koeleria macrantha*	≤10 (NEG)
	Festuca pratensis	≤10 (NEG)
	Dactylis glomerata	≤10 (NEG)
	Lolium perenne	≤10 (NEG)
	Agrostis gigantea	≤10 (NEG)
	Phleum pratense	≤10 (NEG)
	Anthoxanthum odoratum	≤10 (NEG)
	Bromus	≤10 (NEG)
	Oat pollen	≤10 (NEG)
	Sorghum halepense	≤10 (NEG)
	Paspalum notatum	**15 (+)**
	Corn pollen	≤10 (NEG)
	Cynodon dactylon	≤10 (NEG)
Weeds	***Chenopodium berlandieri***	**11 (+)**
	Kochia	**37 (++)**
	Echinops exaltatus	**22 (+)**
	Atriplex	≤10 (NEG)
	Mixed *Ambrosia* (short, tall)	**158 (+++)**
	Franseria acanthicarpa	**90 (+++)**
	Southern ragweed	≤10 (NEG)
	Common ragweed	**125 (+++)**
	Mix of *Salvia* and *Artemisia*	≤10 (NEG)
	Xanthium	≤10 (NEG)
	Iva xanthifolia	≤10 (NEG)
	Iva annua	≤10 (NEG)
	Solidago	≤10 (NEG)
	Eupatorium capillifolium	≤10 (NEG)
	Rumex acetosa	**19 (+)**
	Plantago lanceolata	≤10 (NEG)
	Amaranthus	**14 (+)**
	Nettle	≤10 (NEG)

Trees	**Mix of *Acer negundo***	**13 (+)**
	Mix of oak	≤10 (NEG)
	Beech	≤10 (NEG)
	Mulberry	≤10 (NEG)
	American walnut	≤10 (NEG)
	Pecan	**17 (+)**
	Eastern black walnut	**18 (+)**
	California black walnut	≤10 (NEG)
	Willow	≤10 (NEG)
	Quaking aspen	≤10 (NEG)
	Eastern cottonwood	≤10 (NEG)
	American or white ash	≤10 (NEG)
	Arizona ash	≤10 (NEG)
	Olive	≤10 (NEG)
	Henna	≤10 (NEG)
	Cedar	≤10 (NEG)
	Arizona cypress	≤10 (NEG)
	Bald cypress	≤10 (NEG)
	Mix of elm	**15 (+)**
	Alder	≤10 (NEG)
	Mix of birch	≤10 (NEG)
	Hazelnut	≤10 (NEG)
	Sycamore	≤10 (NEG)
	Acacia	≤10 (NEG)
	Mesquite	**13 (+)**
	Liquidambar	≤10 (NEG)
	Myrtle	≤10 (NEG)
	Pepper tree	≤10 (NEG)
	Mix of pine	≤10 (NEG)
	Queen palm	≤10 (NEG)
	Eucalyptus	≤10 (NEG)
	Melaleuca	≤10 (NEG)
	Australian pine	≤10 (NEG)
Mites	***Dermatophagoides farinae***	**>600 (+++)**
	Dermatophagoides pteronyssinus	**183 (+++)**
	Tyrophagus	**>600 (+++)**
	Acarus siro	**>600 (+++)**
	Lepidoglyphus	**17 (+)**
	Blomia tropicalis	**408 (+++)**

Insects	Flea	≤10 (NEG)
	Mix of cockroaches	≤10 (NEG)
	Mosquito	≤10 (NEG)
Epithelia	Cat	≤10 (NEG)
	Mix of feathers	≤10 (NEG)
Fungi	*Malassezia*	≤10 (NEG)
	Fusarium	**87 (+++)**
	Aspergillus	≤10 (NEG)
	Penicillium	≤10 (NEG)
	Cladosporium	**47 (++)**
	Alternaria	≤10 (NEG)
	Drechslera	≤10 (NEG)
	Mix of wheat blight	**12 (+)**

Allergen-specific IgE serology and intradermal tests yielded positive results for grasses, weeds, trees, dust and storage mites, and fungi. The following information on immunotherapy was given to the client.

Immunotherapy

- Preferable as treatment in non-seasonal cases.
- Allergens selected according to allergy tests and correlated with clinical history.
- The treatment can be given via subcutaneous injections every 10–21 days, or orally once or twice a day.
- Response: ⅓ of patients have a complete response (do not need additional treatment), ⅓ have a partial response (need additional treatments), ⅓ do not respond to the treatment.
- The response cannot be predicted.
- Response depends on:
  - The diagnostic accuracy of the tests.
  - The formulation of the vaccine.
  - The adjustment of the dose and the frequency for each case.
  - How well the owners follow the treatment.
- Generally, a response is observed after 4–6 months, but can take up to 12 months to manifest.
- If no response is observed after 12 months, the treatment is discontinued.
- The dose and/or frequency need to be monitored and changed as necessary.

Adverse reactions

- Anaphylactic shock is very rare.
- An increase in pruritus is sometimes observed after administration of the allergen. If this happens:
  - Lower the dose.
  - Premedicate with antihistamines 30 minutes before administration.

The owner decided to begin treatment with an oral vaccine given twice a day. A follow-up appointment was recommended at 3 months, 6 months and 1 year to evaluate the response.

CONCLUSION

After one year of treatment, Pepe showed a partial response to immunotherapy and only required occasional treatment with oclacitinib, during the spring and autumn. He did not have clinical lesions or secondary infections after starting the treatment. A blood count, chemistry profile and urinalysis were recommended every 6 months to monitor possible side effects of the treatment with oclacitinib, which can cause a decrease in the leukocyte count (neutrophils, monocytes), especially when given at a higher than recommended dose.

The patient's prognosis is good with continued immunotherapy.

If oclacitinib side effects are observed, other options for the most critical months will be discussed, such as the use of glucocorticoids or anti-IL-31 monoclonal antibodies.

PEMPHIGUS FOLIACEUS

Pemphigus foliaceus (PF) is an autoimmune disorder characterised by the presence of pustules and scabs, normally located on the pinnae, the dorsal part of the nose, the foot pads and the nail area in cats. Cytology in these cases reveals the presence of acantholytic keratinocytes, that is, keratinocytes that have lost intercellular adhesion (desmosomes) and are the target of the generated antibodies. Even though acantholytic keratinocytes are distinctive of PF, they are not pathognomonic and may be found in suppurative diseases such as pyoderma and dermatophytosis caused by species of the genus *Tricophyton*. The diagnosis is based on histopathology and on ruling out the previously mentioned diseases. Histopathology reveals subcorneal pustules with the presence of neutrophils and acantholytic keratinocytes. The treatment is based on immunosuppressant drugs, which have shown to be effective against this disease. These drugs include corticosteroids, chlorambucil and cyclosporine as a single or combined treatment

Most patients require a lifelong treatment to maintain the disease in remission.

CLINICAL CASE. BABY GIRL

Mixed domestic shorthair cat, spayed, 6 years old.

PATIENT HISTORY

The patient presented with a 4-day history of lack of energy and development of scaly lesions on her face, ears and paws. Her consumption of food and water was normal. Baby Girl was the only cat in the household. The owners also had two Chihuahuas, but neither the dogs nor the owners had skin lesions.

GENERAL PHYSICAL EXAMINATION

During the physical examination, Baby Girl was alert. Her hydration, temperature, and respiratory and heart rates were normal. She did not present with any abnormalities on abdominal palpation or chest auscultation. She weighed 3.4 kg and her body condition score was 4 out of 9 (thin).

DERMATOLOGICAL EXAMINATION

Yellowish-brown scabs were observed on the dorsal part of the nose, the temporal area, the edge of the inner pinna and the dorsal part of the head (Fig. 1). The outer pinna had diffuse yellowish scabs that extended to the dorsal part of the neck and the trunk.

The border of the scabs on the trunk was associated with erythema (Figs. 2 and 3.) The nail area presented with brown scabs lightly adhered to the skin (Fig. 4).

If acantholytic keratinocytes are observed in the cytological examination, the presence of pyoderma and dermatophytosis caused by species of the genus *Tricophyton* must be ruled out via bacterial and fungal cultures.

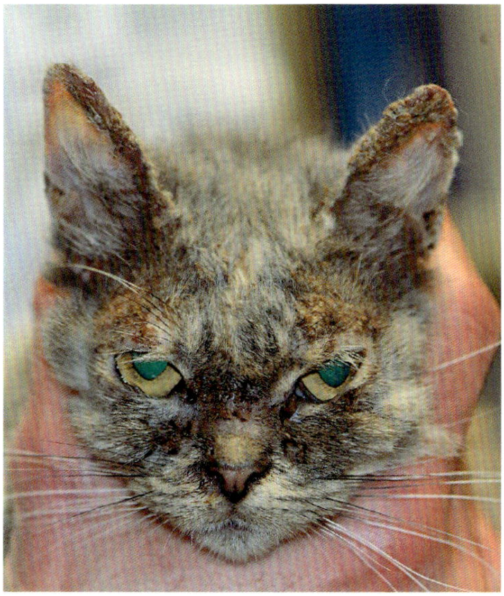

Figure 1. Lesions characteristic of PF: yellowish-brown scabs.

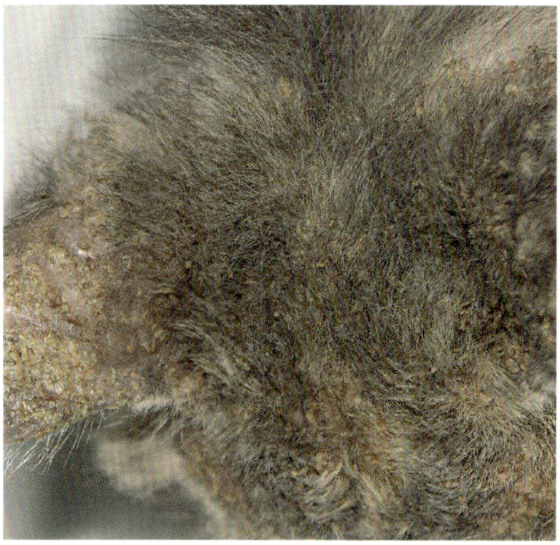

Figure 2. The pinna is frequently affected in cases of PF.

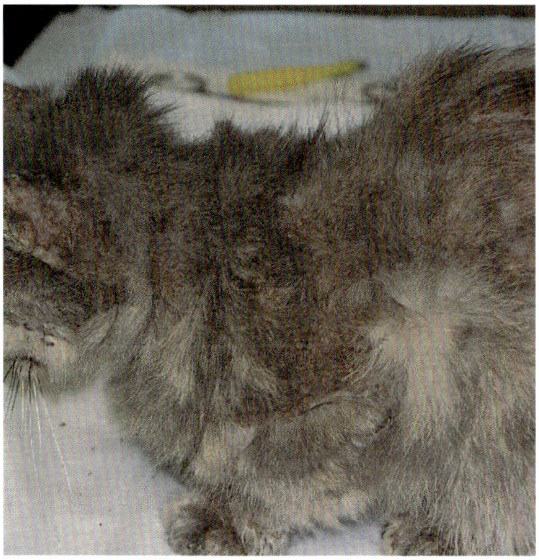

Figure 3. In this case, the trunk is affected since it is a generalised presentation.

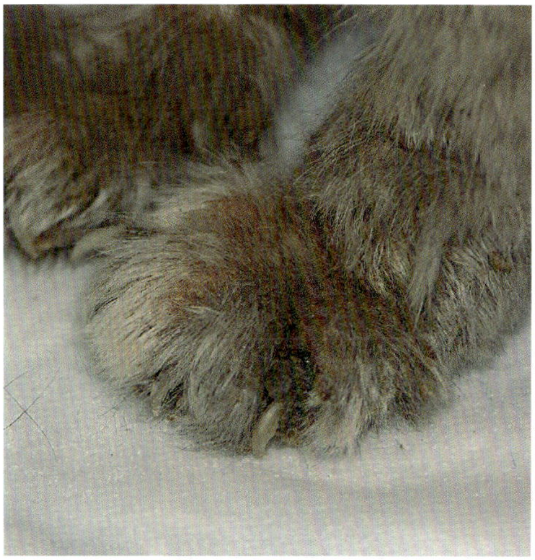

Figure 4. The nail area is frequently affected in cases of feline PF.

DIFFERENTIAL DIAGNOSIS

PF, dermatophytosis and bacterial pyoderma were considered the most likely differential diagnoses. Demodicosis, pemphigus erythematosus, and reaction to medication were also included.

DIAGNOSTIC TESTS AND RESULTS

During the first visit, it was decided to perform a cytological examination after removing a scab and making an impression smear of the exposed area. A hair sample was also taken so it could be examined for spores or hyphae.

The cytological examination revealed the presence of many neutrophils and acantholytic keratinocytes (Fig. 5). No spores or hyphae were observed in the hair sample.

A blood count, chemistry profile and urinalysis were performed. The haematocrit showed leukocytosis with mild neutrophilia. No other significant changes were seen.

According to the differential diagnosis and cytology results, it was decided to take two samples for bacterial and dermatophyte culture. The sample for bacterial culture was taken with a sterile cotton swab from the area under a scab, while the sample for dermatophyte culture included hair and scabs from the external pinna. In addition, a biopsy was taken to perform a histopathological study. The area under one of the chest scabs was infiltrated with 0.5 ml of 2 % lidocaine. After 5 minutes, the sample was taken with a 6-mm punch. The area was sutured with polyglactin 910.

Both cultures were negative and the histopathological examination was consistent with PF (Fig. 6), thereby confirming the diagnosis.

Diagnosis of pemphigus foliaceus

Presence of pustules, yellowish scabs, and erosions that affect primarily the pinnae, face, and paws.

The lesions are generally symmetrical and localised, though they can become generalised.

Cytology reveals acantholytic keratinocytes and neutrophils. In some cases it is also possible to observe a significant number of eosinophils.

Pyoderma and dermatophytosis are important differential diagnoses that must be ruled out.

The definitive diagnosis is based on histopathology.

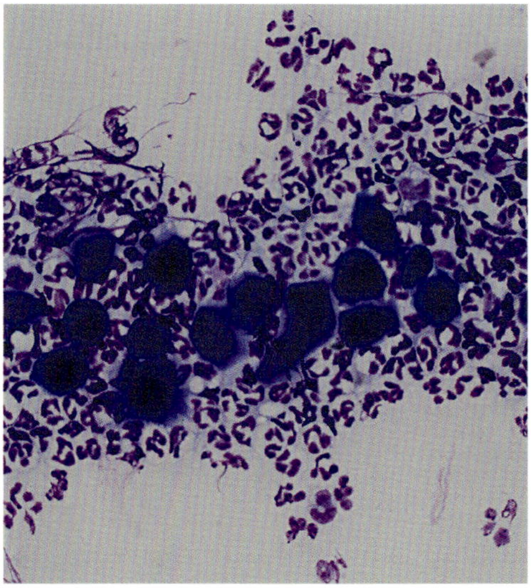

Figure 5. Presence of abundant neutrophils and acantholytic keratinocytes. Cytological image characteristic of PF.

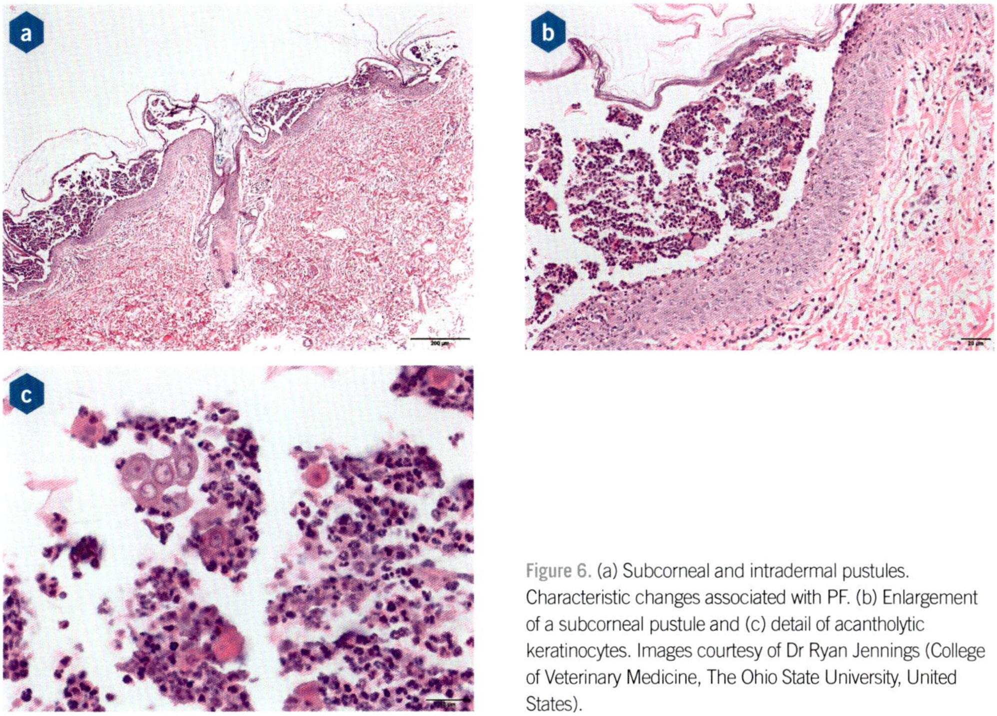

Figure 6. (a) Subcorneal and intradermal pustules. Characteristic changes associated with PF. (b) Enlargement of a subcorneal pustule and (c) detail of acantholytic keratinocytes. Images courtesy of Dr Ryan Jennings (College of Veterinary Medicine, The Ohio State University, United States).

TREATMENT

The treatment of PF includes immunosuppressive doses of glucocorticoids in different options: prednisolone (starting dose: 2–4 mg/kg), triamcinolone (starting dose: 0.4–2 mg/kg), methylprednisolone (starting dose: 1.5–3 mg/kg), dexamethasone (0.2–0.4 mg/kg). The starting dose is maintained until the lesions subside, according to the clinical examination and cytology results (absence of acantholytic cells). The dose of glucocorticoids is then reduced until reaching the minimum dose that maintains the clinical signs in remission. Treatment with prednisolone was started at 2.2 mg/kg (7.5 mg) every 24 hours and cephalosporin at 25 mg/kg every 12 hours. Treatment with cephalosporin was started because a positive correlation has been observed between the use of antibiotics during immunosuppression and patient survival. A follow-up visit 2 weeks after beginning the treatment was recommended.

During the second visit, an improvement of 80 % was observed. The clinical examination only revealed areas of alopecia and flaking in areas previously covered with scabs. The prednisolone dose was lowered to 1.5 mg/kg (5 mg) every 24 hours and treatment with cephalexin was continued until the following appointment 2 weeks later, in which notable improvement was observed. Thus, it was decided to reduce the prednisolone dose to 0.9 mg/kg (3 mg) every 24 hours and to discontinue the treatment with cephalosporin.

Treatment alternatives

If treatment with prednisolone is initiated as a single therapy and the dose cannot be decreased in a way that does not cause significant side effects, treatment with another glucocorticoid or drug may be initiated to reduce the dose of the glucocorticoids used. The following medications can be used as alternatives: triamcinolone (0.4–2 mg/kg every 24 hours), dexamethasone (0.2–0.4 mg/kg every 24 hours), methylprednisolone (1.6–4.8 mg/kg every 24 hours), chlorambucil (0.1–0.2 mg/kg every 24 hours), or cyclosporine (5–10 mg/kg every 24 hours). Side effects derived from the use of chlorambucil include medullary aplasia (anaemia, thrombocytopaenia, panleukopaenia) and gastric problems (vomiting, diarrhoea, anorexia). A blood count is recommended every 15 days and a chemistry profile every 4 weeks for the first 6 months, and then every 3 months thereafter. Side effects from the use of cyclosporine include vomiting, diarrhoea, anorexia, and acute toxoplasmosis. In this case, it is recommended that a blood count, chemistry profile, urinalysis, and urine culture be performed every 6 months. Likewise, it is recommended to measure *Toxoplasma* titres before starting the treatment and to minimise the risk of infection during cyclosporine therapy, since cats receiving cyclosporine treatment are at risk of developing fatal systemic toxoplasmosis.

CONCLUSION

Baby Girl continued with periodic follow-up visits every 4 weeks for the first 6 months. The prednisolone dose was gradually decreased down to 0.3 mg/kg (1 mg) every 48 hours. It was recommended that a blood count, chemistry profile, urinalysis and urine culture be performed every 6 months. The results obtained from these tests after 6 months were within normal limits. The owner was explained that the prognosis for PF is relatively good if the patient continues to tolerate the treatment well, but that most patients require immunosuppressive therapy for life, with the exception of some cases of pemphigus induced by a reaction to medication, in which cases the treatment can eventually be discontinued.

Adjusting the dose of corticosteroids

A starting dose is administered daily until the clinical signs resolve, which generally takes 2–4 weeks. If the clinical signs do not resolve during this period, treatment with another glucocorticoid or other drug may be initiated to decrease the dose of the glucocorticoids used (e.g. chlorambucil or cyclosporine).

When the lesions have resolved, the dose must be decreased gradually, e.g. 25 % every 1–2 weeks, and the patient evaluated every 10–15 days. If there is no relapse, try to reach a dose below 0.5 mg/kg of prednisolone or methylprednisolone every 48 hours.

The maintenance dose of dexamethasone is 0.05 mg/kg every 72 hours, while for triamcinolone it is 0.1 mg/kg every 72 hours.

CHRONIC RECURRENT OTITIS

The successful management of otitis externa requires a complete clinical history and physical examination. Most patients with otitis externa present with head shaking and pruritus, and their owners note the presence of exudate and/or of an unpleasant odour. Animals with otitis media or interna develop other, different clinical signs (Table 1). Otitis externa can be a recurring problem. It has been noted that 82 % of chronic cases were associated with otitis media. The clinical history can be crucial to establish the primary cause, and any clinical abnormalities can provide additional information (e.g. presence of pruritus in other areas or gastrointestinal signs that can suggest an underlying allergy). Otoscopic examination while the patient is awake is usually limited by patient tolerance and the presence of exudate in the ear canal.

Frequently, otitis is very painful and patients do not permit the otoscopic examination without sedation or anesthesia.

The goal of the otoscopic examination is to identify foreign bodies, ulcers (usually seen in infections caused by *Pseudomonas*), hyperplasia, tumours, and, ideally, to evaluate the eardrum, which may be damaged in cases of otitis media.

Table 1. Clinical signs of otitis externa, media, and interna.

Otitis externa	Otitis media	Otitis interna

▸ Head shaking.
▸ Pruritus.
▸ Ear alopecia.
▸ Excoriated ear flaps.
▸ Exudate in the ear canal.
▸ Unpleasant odour.
▸ Pain.
▸ Behavioural changes.
	▸ Recurrent otitis externa.
	▸ Facial nerve paralysis.
	  ▸ Facial asymmetry.
	  ▸ Drooping ear flap.
	  ▸ Sialorrhea.
	  ▸ Eyelid areflexia.
	  ▸ Keratoconjunctivitis sicca
	▸ Horner's syndrome:
	  ▸ Protrusion of the third eyelid.
	  ▸ Enophthalmos.
	  ▸ Miosis.
	  ▸ Ptosis.
		▸ Horizontal nystagmus.
		▸ Head tilt.
		▸ Body instability towards the affected side, walking in circles.
		▸ Ataxia.

CLINICAL CASE. TARA

Female scent hound, spayed, 5 years old.

PATIENT HISTORY

The patient had been suffering from chronic recurrent otitis for 3 years. During this time, Tara had received several treatments, including topical and systemic drugs. The most recent treatment had been administered 1 month before the appointment and consisted in the application of a topical treatment containing enrofloxacin 0.23 %, ketoconazole 1 %, and triamcinolone 0.1 % in a lanolin base. The owners had not noted any improvement and thought that Tara did not hear well after the treatment. The patient continued to scratch and had an unpleasant odour in her ears. Although both ears were affected, the right ear was more severely damaged. The clinical signs were present year round, but the owners thought that the problem was worse in spring and autumn, seasons in which she also licked her paws. Their veterinary surgeon had recently prescribed oclacitinib, which had improved the pruritus in her paws, but not in her ears. Tara was fed a diet based on salmon and potatoes.

GENERAL PHYSICAL EXAMINATION

During the physical examination, Tara was alert. Her hydration, temperature, heart rhythm and rate and respiratory rate were normal. Her lung sounds were clear; no heart murmur was heard. The patient was ambulatory and had no weakness or ataxia; her behaviour was normal. No lymphadenopathy was noted, although moderate dental calculus was observed.

DERMATOLOGICAL EXAMINATION

Slight erythema was noted on the chin and perivulvar area. The pinna of the right ear had moderate erythema and a yellowish-white exudate was observed. The rest of the dermatological examination was normal. It was not possible to perform an otoscopic examination due to pain and the presence of exudate.

DIFFERENTIAL DIAGNOSIS

Allergic dermatitis was considered as the underlying cause of the recurrent otitis. Since there was a history of seasonality, atopic dermatitis was considered, but the possibility of a multiple aetiology was not ruled out. Since the dog was a scent hound, the structure of the ear and pinnae was also taken into account as risk factors.

DIAGNOSTIC TESTS AND RESULTS

Samples were taken from the ear canals for a cytological examination during the first visit. No organisms or inflammatory cells were found in the sample from the left ear, but a large number of bacilli and the occasional presence of cocci were observed in the sample from the right ear. The exudate also included inflammatory cells, primarily neutrophils and, in smaller numbers, lymphocytes and macrophages (Fig. 1).

Otitis externa was diagnosed based on the cytological findings and clinical signs.

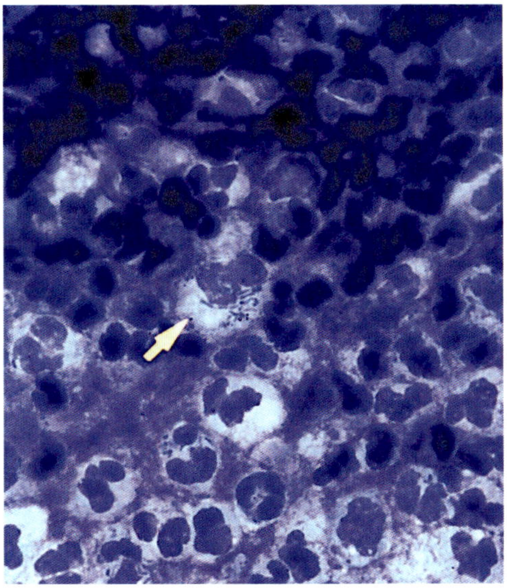

Figure 1. The sample from the right ear canal had a large number of bacilli and occasional cocci.

Given the chronic problem and the possible presence of otitis media as a perpetuating factor for otitis externa, computed tomography (CT) was recommended to assess the middle ear. At the same time, with the patient under general anaesthesia, the ear is also washed and the ear canal assessed with a video otoscope. When exudate is present in the middle ear, a myringotomy is performed (see *Miringotomy*, pages 26 and 27) to take a sample from the middle ear and flush the tympanic bulla.

It was discussed whether a CT scan would be performed instead of X-rays, as it can be difficult to position the patient and interpret the findings in radiographic examinations of the bullae; 25 % of dogs with otitis media do not present significant radiographic changes.

A blood sample was taken to perform a blood count as well as a chemistry profile to obtain baseline values before starting treatment and decide on the best anaesthesia protocol.

TREATMENT

Oral prednisone (0.9 mg/kg daily) was prescribed until the second visit (for CT and ear lavage), which was scheduled to take place 2 weeks later. Prednisone is indicated to reduce inflammation, pain and the amount of exudate in the ear canal. The use of oclacitinib was not recommended, since no studies have evaluated the safety of these treatments when administered together.

The owners were informed of the likelihood of allergic dermatitis being the primary cause of the recurrent otitis and it was decided to begin an elimination diet to diagnose or rule out a possible food intolerance. A kangaroo and oat–based diet was started.

An appointment was made for 2 weeks later to perform the CT and ear lavage under general anaesthesia. The owners were asked not to feed Tara after 10 pm the day before the second visit.

Follow-up

A general examination was performed that did not reveal any abnormalities. The total protein (6.8 g/dl) and haematocrit (43 %) values were within normal ranges. Tara was premedicated with dexmedetomidine and intramuscular morphine, and anaesthesia was induced with intravenous propofol and maintained with isoflurane gas.

Keeping the ear clean and open, using the appropriate antibiotics, and frequent follow-up visits are critical issues to consider when managing recurrent otitis.

Myringotomy

If otitis media is suspected in a patient, a myringotomy (incision in the tympanic membrane) may be a useful diagnostic test to help confirm the presence of fluid in the middle ear and collect a sample for bacterial culture. A myringotomy can also be therapeutic, as it relieves pressure in the middle ear and allows the exudate to be flushed away. Ideally, the presence of fluid in the middle ear should be confirmed by CT. Figure 2 shows fluid in both tympanic bullae, with a greater amount in the right one. The availability and cost of CT can be prohibitive for some clients. It has been shown that radiography is not as reliable and accurate as CT. A study comparing CT with surgical histopathology of otitis media found that the former had a sensitivity of 86 % and a specificity of 89 % (Remedios et al, 1991). Ultrasound whas been used as an alternative to CT. Magnetic resonance imaging, which has a sensitivity of 80–100 % and a specificity of 74–100 %, can also be used for the detection of fluid.

Equipment needed:

- Video otoscope.
- 5-Fr urinary catheter.
- Sterile container for bacterial culture sample.
- Warm sterile saline solution.
- Bulb syringe.
- 6-ml syringes.

First, the ear canal must be cleaned. The incision should be made in the caudoventral quadrant of the pars tensa with the 5-Fr urinary catheter. If the manubrium (one of the ossicles in the middle ear) is observed, avoid touching it with the catheter. If it cannot be seen (due to fluids or masses in the middle ear or thickening of the tympanic membrane), avoid touching the dorsal rostral area of the tympanic membrane to minimise damage to the ossicles.

Sometimes the tympanic membrane is already torn, or is not present, and the tympanic bulla can be seen directly. If it is already torn in the correct area to perform the myringotomy, samples can be obtained and cleaning performed through the existing tear. If the tear is not in the correct area, it is recommended to perform the myringotomy in the correct area.

Using sterile scissors, 7–10 inches should be cut from the tip of the rigid sterile catheter at a 60-degree angle, leaving 12–15 inches of catheter with a sharp tip. This catheter is then fed through the port of the otoscope until it is just in front of the tympanic membrane. With a firm movement, the catheter is pushed through the tympanic membrane (Fig. 3). Sometimes fluid or debris from the bulla come out of the incision.

With a syringe and a new sterile catheter, the middle ear fluid should be aspirated and retained for a cytological examination and culture. If no fluid is present, 0.5–1 ml of sterile saline is injected into the middle ear and aspirated to collect a sample for culture.

The bulla is then gently rinsed with warm sterile saline solution, between 10 and 20 times (approximately 60–120 ml total saline) until no more debris or opaque fluid comes out of the bulla and the bone of the bulla can be felt with the catheter (the catheter rubs against something hard and gritty). Care must be taken not to rinse with too much pressure, as further tearing of the tympanic membrane may occur. If the tympanic membrane is accidentally torn, it heals within 21–28 days. All the fluid in the bulla and the ear canal is then aspirated.

Rarely, patients will develop vestibular signs after the procedure. This is usually temporary and can be treated as needed, usually with systemic glucocorticoids and antiemetics, based on the severity.

Finally, the samples are sent for bacterial culture.

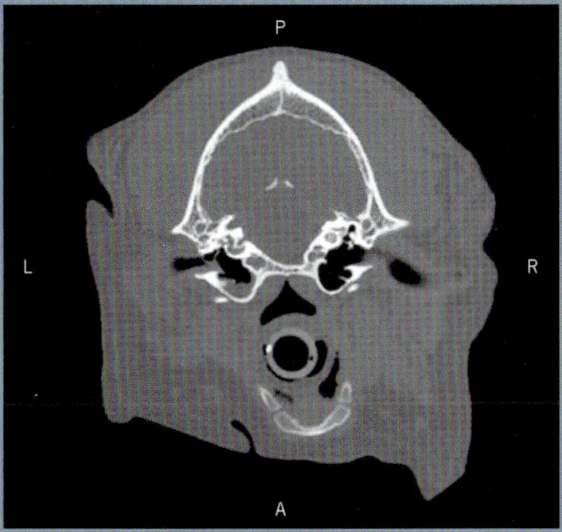

Figure 2. CT of a patient with unilateral otitis media.

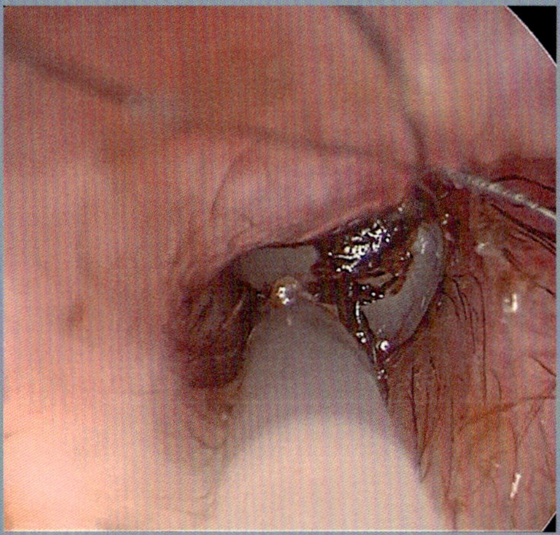

Figure 3. Catheter going through the tympanic membrane in the posterior ventral quadrant during a myringotomy.

Computed tomography

Both tympanic bullae were filled with air and no bone changes were observed. Mild cartilage mineralisation was seen in both ear canals, which showed an increase in density consistent with the presence of exudate or soft tissue. Isohexol was administered intravenously as a contrast agent. No raised areas were observed, so the presence of a tumour was ruled out. The retropharyngeal lymph nodes were of normal size (Fig. 4).

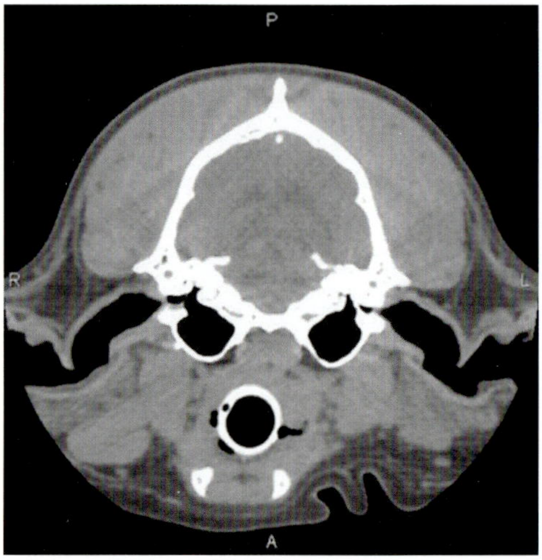

Figure 4. Tara's CT scan. Both tympanic bullae were filled with air, free of exudate.

Video otoscope examination and ear lavage

Slight erythema was observed in the horizontal and vertical canals of the left ear. A moderate amount of exudate and fat was found in the ear canal. After manually flushing the canal with warm saline solution and a bulb syringe, further cleaning was performed under video-otoscopic guidance. A 5-Fr catheter was inserted through the opening of the video otoscope and the ear was cleaned with the aid of a suction pump. Once the ear canal was cleaned, the tympanic membrane, which was intact and normal in thickness and colour, could be observed.

The right ear canal had moderate erythema and an abundant amount of ceruminous exudate in the lumen and adhered to the wall of the canal. The canal was flushed with warm saline solution, as described for the left ear, and the tympanic membrane was assessed, showing no rupture or changes in colour and structure (Fig. 5).

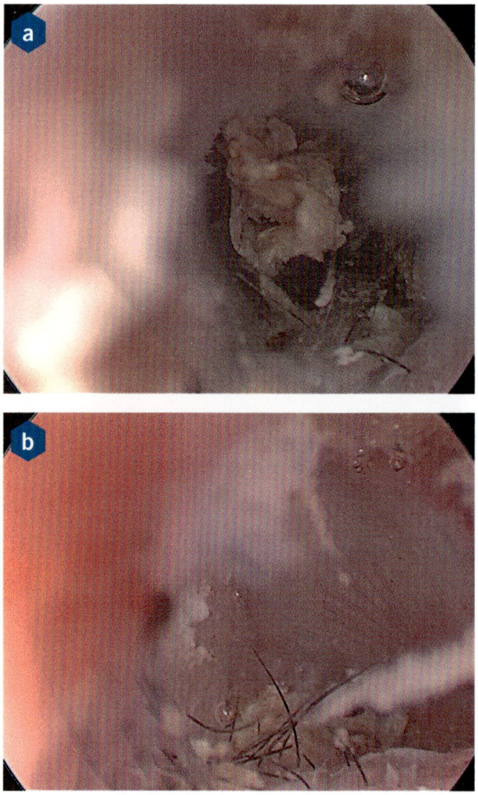

Figure 5. Right ear canal (a) before and (b) after lavage.

Cytology

Samples from both ear canals were taken for a cytological examination and culture using sterile swabs. No organisms or inflammatory cells were present in the left canal. The right canal, on the other hand, had a considerable number of bacilli and occasional yeasts; the exudate also included inflammatory cells, mainly neutrophils and, to a lesser extent, lymphocytes and macrophages. Samples of exudate from the right ear canal were sent for bacterial culture.

Treatment after bacterial culture

Treatment with oral prednisone was discontinued as the patient had developed polyuria and intense polydipsia.

The bacterial culture results indicated the presence of *Pseudomonas aeruginosa* and *Escherichia coli*. Both organisms are susceptible to fluoroquinolones, so the following treatment protocol was established:

1. Flush both ears with a neutral pH solution twice a week. The owner was given written instructions on how to do the cleaning.
2. One millilitre of a tri-EDTA solution (pretreatment) was administered in the right ear twice a day, 15 minutes before applying enrofloxacin drops.
3. One millilitre of an enrofloxacin-silver sulfadiazine solution was administered in the right ear twice a day.
4. Immediately after the enrofloxacin solution, 0.5 ml of miconazole (1 % solution) was applied to the right ear twice a day.

The owners were encouraged to continue the elimination diet begun after the previous appointment.

An appointment was made for the patient 2 weeks later. A cytological examination was performed during the follow-up visit and was negative in both ears. The owner was told to continue the treatments for 2 weeks, until the next appointment. At week 4 of treatment, the cytology results remained negative and a sample was taken for bacterial culture. The owner was instructed to continue the treatment as indicated above.

The bacterial culture was negative, so the treatment was discontinued after 5 weeks of topical treatment and 7 weeks of elimination diet.

After 12 weeks of elimination diet, the patient was examined and a cytological examination of samples collected from both ear canals yielded negative results. It was decided to discontinue the elimination diet and resume the previous diet. Four days after the diet change, Tara started scratching her ears. A short treatment with oral prednisone (1 mg/kg/day for 3 days) was prescribed and the kangaroo-based diet was resumed.

CONCLUSION

Tara continued with weekly ear flushing, a kangaroo-based diet and oclacitinib during spring and autumn to relieve the pruritus of the limbs.

> The prognosis of patients with chronic otitis depends on their response to the treatment and on the possibility of identifying and controlling primary, perpetuating, and risk factors.

If the ear canals are not opened with glucocorticoids or if infections are still present after prolonged topical treatments and systemic antimicrobial treatments, it is very difficult to continue to handle the case medically. If this point is reached, the best option is a total ablation of the ear canal and an osteotomy of the tympanic bulla. Fortunately, that course is not often necessary with a proper therapy and management.

Successful treatment of otitis caused by *Pseudomonas* can be a challenge, but it is usually resolved through appropriate management.

HEPATOCUTANEOUS SYNDROME

(necrolytic migratory erythema, metabolic epidermal necrosis, superficial necrolytic dermatitis)

Necrolytic migratory erythema is the term used in human medicine to describe skin lesions associated with glucagonomas (pancreatic tumours that secrete glucagon) or cirrhosis of the liver. Similar lesions have been described in dogs and cats, but are more commonly associated with liver disease. Only a minority of the cases described in veterinary medicine correspond to glucagonomas. Diseases that have been associated with superficial necrolytic dermatitis in dogs include glucagon-producing pancreatic endocrine tumours, hyperglucagonaemia and glucagon-secreting hepatic metastases (primary tumour not found), gastrointestinal disease (vomiting, diarrhoea), liver disease secondary to the ingestion of mycotoxins, liver disease secondary to the administration of phenobarbital/phenytoin sodium, copper-associated liver disease, and idiopathic liver disease.

Hypoaminoacidaemia and/or deficiency of biotin, zinc, and essential fatty acids have been proposed as the cause of the skin lesions.

Hypoaminoacidaemia may also be responsible for hepatic changes. This claim is based in part on the fact that, when fed a protein-deficient diet for prolonged periods of time, dogs develop hypoalbuminaemia and liver changes that resemble those described in the hepatocutaneous syndrome, although no skin lesions are observed. The importance of hypoaminoacidaemia in this disease is further supported by the fact that the administration of intravenous amino acid solutions temporarily improves skin lesions in many, but not all, dogs. The cause of the amino acid deficiency is unknown. Most affected dogs are fed diets with an adequate protein content.

Although in some cases liver disease has been associated with the presence of toxins and the use of anticonvulsive drugs, most cases are idiopathic.

Any breed can be affected. However, it was recently described in a group of 31 Shih Tzus, so a possible hereditary predisposition in this

This syndrome generally occurs in older dogs.

breed has been proposed. The lesions are scaly with erosions or ulcerations. The most affected regions are the muzzle, mucocutaneous areas, paws including foot pads, mouth, elbows, genitals and abdomen. Blood tests may show normocytic, normochromic nonregenerative anaemia, hyperglycaemia, elevated liver enzymes and hypoalbuminaemia. The abdominal ultrasound shows a pathognomonic pattern that resembles a "honeycomb". Histopathology of the skin shows parakeratosis, vacuolation of the keratinocytes of the upper layers and hyperplasia, which gives it a characteristic appearance that has been described as "the French flag" (red, white and blue).

CLINICAL CASE. OREO

Male chocolate Labrador, neutered, 11 years old.

PATIENT HISTORY

The patient had a clinical history of 4 months of scaly skin lesions, which had initially affected the face, elbows, and more recently the paws. All this caused Oreo to present with lack of energy, loss of appetite and pain when walking. After a first visit to his veterinary surgeon, he had been prescribed prednisolone for 3 weeks, which had improved the lesions, although they had reappeared once the treatment had been discontinued. Prednisone had then been prescribed, but the clinical signs had not improved. The only treatment the patient was receiving at the time of the appointment was a liver protector containing SAMe (S-adenosyl methionine) and silybin, as the chemistry profile performed by his vet showed increased levels of the enzymes alanine aminotransferase (ALT), gamma glutamyl transpeptidase (GGT), and alkaline phosphatase (ALP).

GENERAL PHYSICAL EXAMINATION

During the general physical examination, Oreo was calm but alert. His hydration and temperature were normal. His heart rate was 88 beats per minute and his respiratory rate was 24 breaths per minute. A mild generalised lymphadenopathy was observed, along with mucopurulent exudate in both eyes.

DERMATOLOGICAL EXAMINATION

The examination revealed severe erythema on the nose and fissures in the upper lips (Fig. 1); erosion/ulceration on the lateral canthus of both eyes (Fig. 2); ulcerative lesions on the elbows (Fig. 3); hyperkeratosis, scabs, and fissures in the plantar pads; intense erythema of the interplantar (Fig. 4) and interdigital areas; and scabbing and erythema in the perianal area.

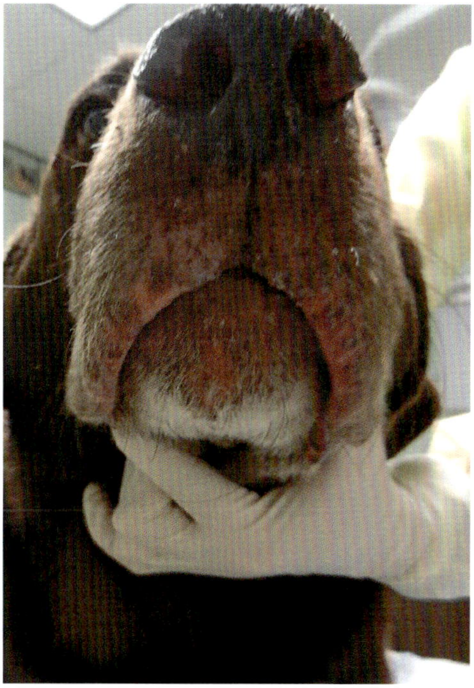

Figure 1. Severe erythema and fissures in the upper lips.

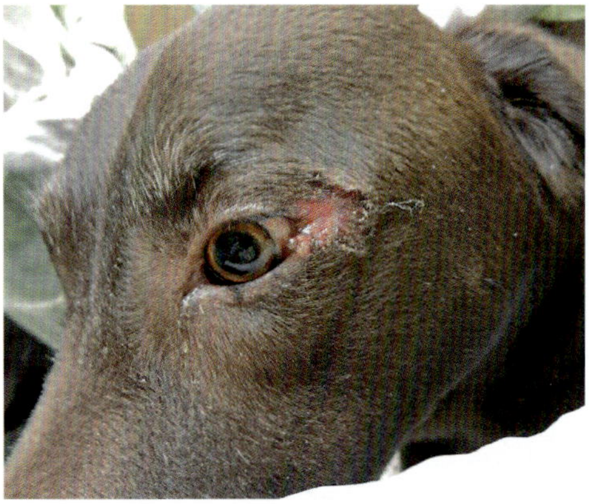

Figure 2. Ulcerative lesion on the lateral canthus of the eye.

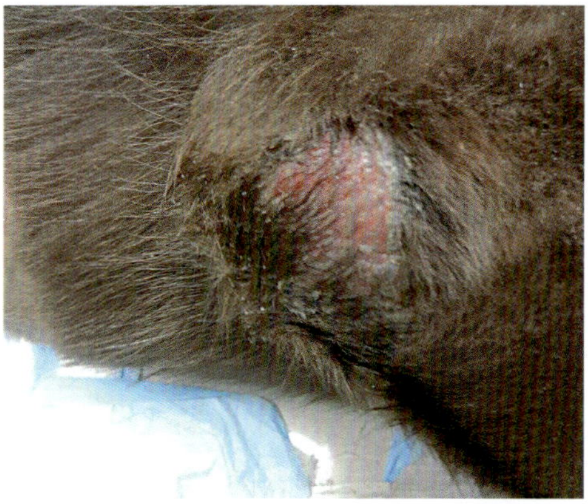

Figure 3. Ulcerative/scaly lesions on the right elbow.

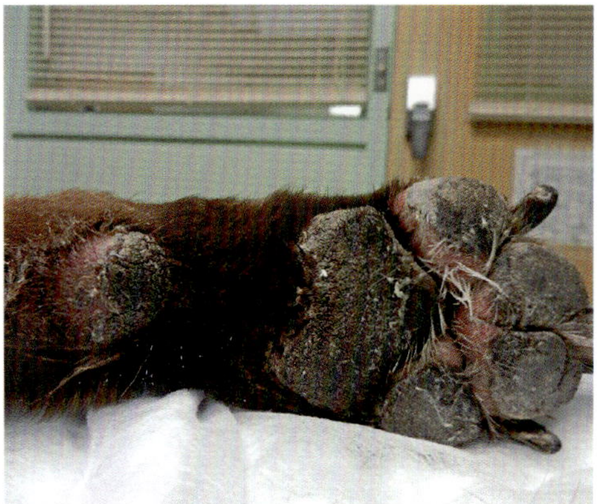

Figure 4. Hyperkeratosis, scabs and fissures in the plantar pads, and intense erythema of the interplantar and interdigital areas.

DIFFERENTIAL DIAGNOSIS

In this case, the importance of the skin lesions cannot be underestimated. Diseases that cause ulcerative/erosive lesions, including plantar pad lesions, along with systemic signs, make cutaneous manifestations of a systemic disease move to the top of the list of differential diagnoses. As the list of systemic diseases that can lead to skin lesions is not very extensive, the differential diagnosis included hepatocutaneous syndrome, zinc-responsive dermatosis, cutaneous lymphoma and, although less likely due to the distribution and presence of ulcers, pemphigus foliaceus.

DIAGNOSTIC TESTS AND RESULTS

It was decided to perform a cytological examination of the skin lesions to identify the presence of inflammatory cells, neoplastic cells, and/or secondary infections. An abdominal ultrasound was also performed. A blood chemistry profile was not repeated, as Oreo's usual vet had performed this test recently.

The cytological examination of the skin showed neutrophils and a significant number of coccoid bacteria, which are findings consistent with superficial pyoderma.

The abdominal ultrasound showed a slight increase in the liver size, a heterogeneous echotexture and the presence of multiple hypoechoic areas and diffuse heterogeneity of the liver parenchyma. These changes gave the liver a "honeycomb" appearance (Fig. 5). A liver aspirate was performed, which showed mild hepatocellular atypia.

When the ultrasound is not diagnostic or is unavailable, a skin biopsy is indicated to confirm the diagnosis. Since the histopathological changes of the hepatocutaneous syndrome are very characteristic and allow a diagnosis to be established, taking the biopsy from a

Hepatocutaneous syndrome was diagnosed based on the clinical signs, the chemistry profile and the results obtained from the abdominal ultrasound and liver aspirate.

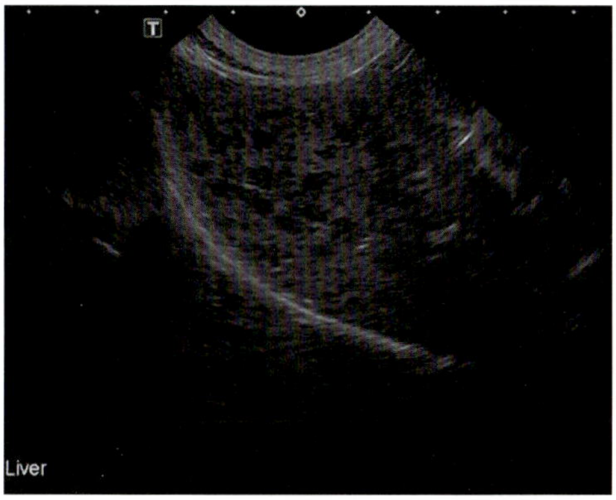

Figure 5. Abdominal ultrasound. Abdominal cranial view showing the pathognomonic "honeycomb" pattern of the liver.

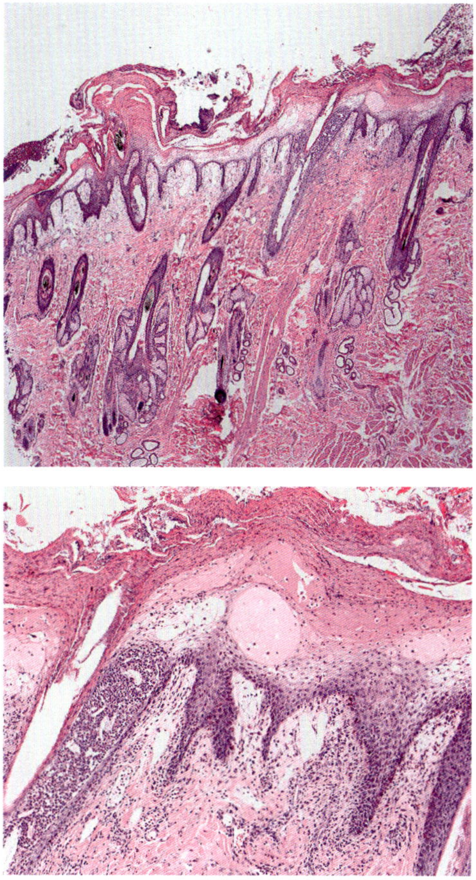

Figure 6. Histopathological image characteristic of the hepatocutaneous syndrome. Hyperplastic epidermis (blue) with an area of oedema, pallor, or necrosis in the stratum spinosum (white) that underlies parakeratotic hyperkeratosis (red), producing a characteristic red, white and blue appearance. Image courtesy of Dr Ryan Jennings (College of Veterinary Medicine, The Ohio State University, United States).

nonulcerated area is recommended, as all the diagnostic changes are in the epidermis (Fig. 6).

TREATMENT

The skin lesions in this syndrome are indicative of a serious illness with a short survival time. A study showed that most patients die or are euthanised within 5 months of being diagnosed. The management of animals with liver disease is problematic. Skin lesions improve, as initially seen in this case, with glucocorticoids, but these are unfortunately contraindicated as they can lead to a diabetic crisis. If the liver disease is not associated with a toxin or medication, it is usually incurable.

Since the skin lesions are thought to be due to deficiencies in amino acids, zinc, biotin, and essential fatty acids, supplementation may be beneficial. It was recommended to include egg yolk (1 yolk/4.5 kg in weight), zinc sulfate (10 mg/kg/day) and essential fatty acids in the dog's diet.

The following oral medications were also prescribed:

- Amoxicillin (15 mg/kg/12 hours): treatment with amoxicillin was started, since in patients with chronic liver fibrosis there is an increased risk of bacterial translocation (passage of bacteria from the gastrointestinal tract to normally sterile tissues such as the bloodstream).
- Mirtazapine (30 mg/day) to stimulate appetite. An antidepressant that also acts as an appetite stimulant by regulating norepinephrine receptors.
- Lactulose (0.5 mg/kg/12 hours): indicated to reduce ammonia levels in the blood so as to prevent hepatic encephalopathy.

For skin lesions, a topical treatment was established as follows:

- Ophthalmic ointment based on neomycin, bacitracin and polymyxin B: apply a small amount in the area around the eyes every 12 hours.
- Ointment based on gentamicin, clotrimazole and mometasone furoate: apply a small amount to affected areas every 12 hours. The patient should be prevented from licking the ointment for half an hour after its application.

It was recommend to include egg yolks, a zinc supplement and essential fatty acids in Oreo's diet if he began to eat normally, and a commercial diet for liver problems was prescribed.

CONCLUSION

Unfortunately, Oreo's liver disease was advanced and the indicated treatments were only palliative. The owner was given an appointment for 2 weeks later, but came back to the clinic a week after the initial visit, since Oreo had not shown any improvement and his overall condition had worsened. As a result, it was decided to perform euthanasia.

Another treatment alternative includes the use of intravenous amino acids. The solution (8–10 %) is administered in a central vein, at a rate of approximately 60–80 mg/kg/24 hours. Osmolarity and/or neurological signs should be monitored daily for 2–3 days, and the treatment may be repeated every 3–6 weeks.

When treating the underlying disease (drug-induced liver disease, resection of a glucagonoma) and secondary skin infections (bacterial and/or yeast), patients often respond positively for a variable period of time, sometimes for more than a year. If liver disease is advanced, the prognosis becomes worse.

In general, the prognosis for this disease is poor and usually most patients die, either due to liver failure, the severity of the skin lesions, or both.

DEMODICOSIS

Demodicosis is the clinical manifestation that results from an excessive proliferation of mites of the genus *Demodex*, of which several host-specific species have been identified. It is a parasite of mammals transmitted by mothers to their offspring during the first days of life.

In dogs, the most common aetiological agent is *Demodex canis*. Its entire life cycle takes place in the hair follicle.

Another, larger species, possibly an inhabitant of the sebaceous gland, named *D. injai*, and a third species with a short body, presumably an inhabitant of the epidermis, called *D. cornei* have been described. Studies using polymerase chain reaction (PCR) have determined that *D. canis* and *D. cornei* are probably different stages of development of *D. canis*.

Certain dog breeds are predisposed to demodicosis, such as the Shar Pei, the West Higland White Terrier, the English Bulldog, the French Bulldog, the Boxer, and the Pug, while in cats breed predisposition is not clear. There is no sex predilection. It is considered juvenile when it presents before 2 years of age and adult if it begins after that age. In addition, it is classified as localised if the patient presents with four or five well-delimited, small-sized areas, with no tendency to grow and without the appearance of new lesions. When more lesions appear and tend to grow and affect whole regions, it is considered generalised. It is important to note that lesions, regardless of the age of onset and whether they are localised or generalised, may show characteristics of superficial folliculitis (in which case there are lesions such as papules, pustules, erythema, epidermal collarettes, comedones, flaking, hyperpigmentation, and alopecia) or deep folliculitis (in which case, in addition to the above-mentioned lesions, intense swelling, scabs and erosions/ulcers are observed, together with fistulous tracts which drain a significant amount of purulent exudate).

At the moment, research has not been able to clarify the mechanism under which excessive proliferation of the parasite takes place. Many of the proposed disorders, such as deficient production of IL-2 and the greater (more than normal) ratio of CD8+ cells to CD4+ cells, are consequences rather than causes of a massive parasite infestation. However, some findings provide some insight into this. For example, increased levels of IL-10 (or at least of a molecule with a very similar composition and activity) have been found in many cases of generalised demodicosis, which could explain to a large extent the most representative disorder of generalised demodicosis, immune depletion. Immune depletion is defined as the recruitment of large numbers of lymphocytes and inflammatory cells, which make a significant but unsuccessful effort to inactivate the infectious or parasitic agent. As the disease spreads, the amount of cells reaching the inflammation site is lower, as is the ability to inactivate the causative agent. In fact, in cases of generalised demodicosis, immune and inflammatory responses occur without adequate signalling.

Clinical case courtesy of Octavio Mejía Ponce (School of Veterinary Medicine and Animal Husbandry, National Autonomous University of Mexico).

CLINICAL CASE. ZEUS

Male German Shepherd, neutered, 2 years old.

PATIENT HISTORY

The patient was acquired as a puppy. He was fed with a commercial diet and did not have any space restrictions at home. His immunisation schedule and deworming and flea treatment was complete and current at the time of the appointment.

The skin lesions had started to appear when Zeus was a year old. On the advice of their veterinary surgeon, the owners had used amitraz and ivermectin (the latter weekly subcutaneously). As they did not see any improvement, they went to another clinic and treatment with prednisone (10 mg total), due to pruritus, and enrofloxacin (5 mg/kg) was started. Some improvement was initially observed in the patient, but shortly thereafter the lesions spread at a faster rate.

GENERAL PHYSICAL EXAMINATION

During the general physical examination, Zeus was alert. His mucous membranes were hyperaemic; capillary filling time was 1–2 seconds. The swallowing and cough reflexes were retained. The lung fields had no abnormalities and percussion was negative. The patient's heart rate was 100 beats per minute; his respiratory rate was 30 breaths per minute. He presented with generalised lymphadenomegaly. His pulse was strong, full, and regular, and abdominal palpation did not show abnormalities. His body condition was 2 out of 5, and his temperature was 38.2 °C.

DERMATOLOGICAL EXAMINATION

The skin lesions were generalised. They consisted of alopecia, erythema, small papules, and pustules as primary lesions, and alopecia, lichenification, comedones, flaking, scabs, and hyperpigmentation as secondary lesions. Virtually the entire skin surface was affected. Several areas exuded a serosanguinous fluid, the legs being the most affected, with the presence of erosions, ulcers, purulent exudate and scabs (Fig. 1–3).

DIFFERENTIAL DIAGNOSIS

Based on the history and clinical examination, generalised demodicosis, deep pyoderma, and dermatophytosis were considered as the most likely differential diagnoses.

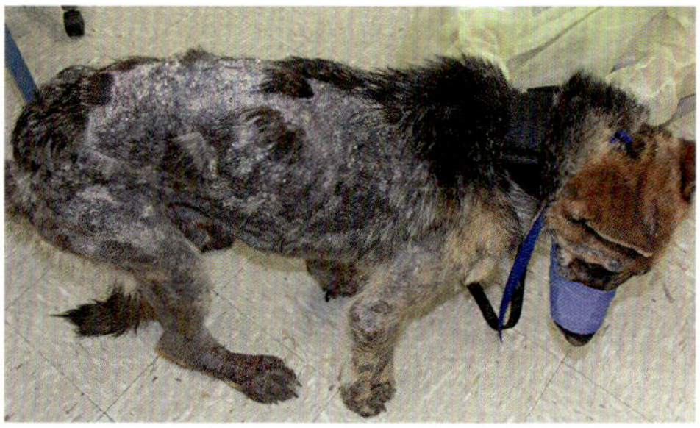

Figure 1. Generalised alopecia, hyperpigmentation, scabs, fistulas and papules.

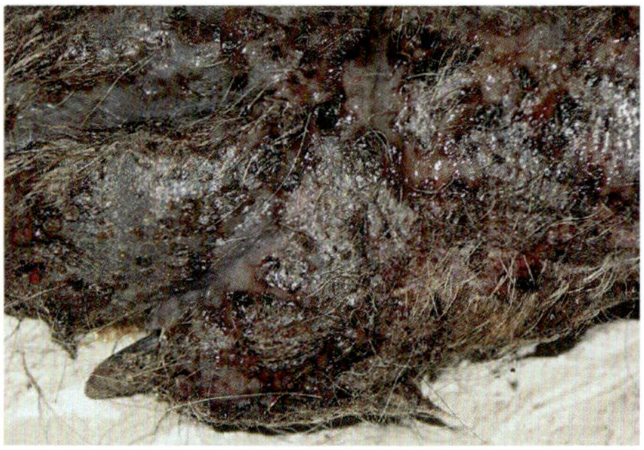

Figure 2. Severe pododermatitis. Alopecia, hyperpigmentation, fistulas, erosions, ulcers and scabs are observed.

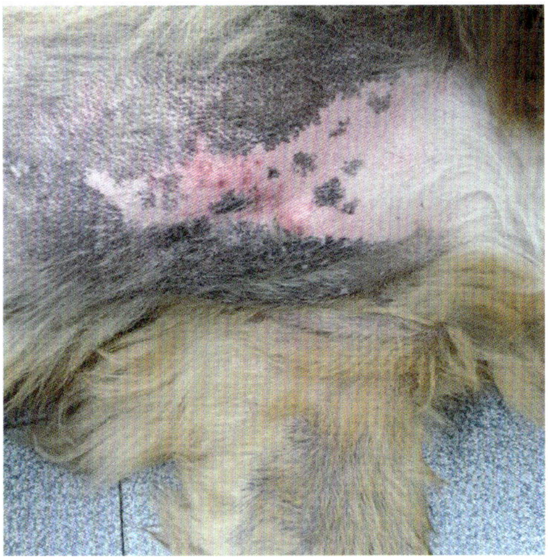

Figure 3. Erythematous papules and comedones are observed on the chest. Hyperpigmentation and hypotrichosis can also be seen on the inner part of the forelimb.

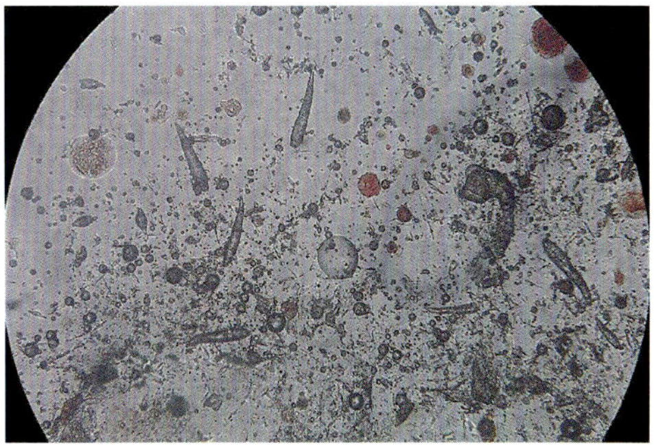

Figure 4. Skin scraping showing adults, nymphs, larvae, and eggs of *Demodex* spp.

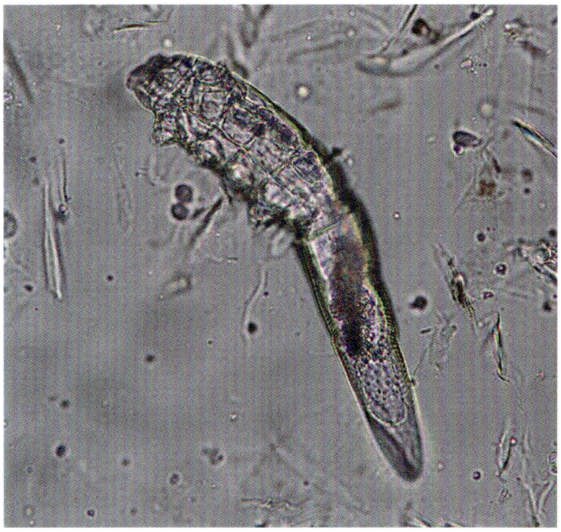

Figure 5. Enlarged image of an adult *D. canis* mite.

DIAGNOSTIC TESTS AND RESULTS

The diagnosis of demodicosis is based on finding the mites that cause demodectic mange by means of deep skin scrapings. It was previously considered indispensable to find juvenile forms of the parasite (eggs, larvae, or nymphs) to obtain a positive diagnosis. Currently, finding a few adult mites in the presence of compatible lesions is considered positive and justifies treatment in cases of generalised presentation.

The microscopic study of a hair sample (tricography) may also be helpful, since it is often possible to find mites in the root of hairs from the affected areas. For its part, histopathology is a very sensitive technique to recognise mites, especially in cases in which scrapings are negative.

From the differential diagnosis it was decided to perform deep scrapings of the affected areas, which were positive for *Demodex canis*. Mites were observed in the different stages of their life cycle (adults and juvenile forms). They were abundant in all the fields **(Figs. 4 and 5)**.

Samples obtained with acetate tape impression and impression smears of exudate were also examined cytologically and showed suppurative inflammation with cocci and macrophages.

Blood samples were also taken for clinical analyses. The results were as follows:

- Blood count: neutrophilic leukocytosis (17.4×10^9/l and 13.0×10^9/l, respectively), regenerative anaemia (haematocrit: 0.31 l/l; erythrocytes: 5.1×10^{12}/l) and an increase in total solids (99 g/l). All of this was a result of the inflammatory process.

- Blood chemistry: prerenal azotaemia (8.1 mmol/l), increased levels of the enzymes alanine aminotranferase (ALT) and alkaline phosphatase (ALP) (202 IU/l and 586 IU/l, respectively), and hyperglobulinaemia (74 g/l). These data were also related to the inflammatory process (hyperglobulinaemia) and dehydration (azotaemia), although this was not clinically evident, in addition to the effect of the administered steroids (increase in ALT and ALP enzymes).

The urinalysis did not show abnormalities.

TREATMENT

The decision to treat a dog with demodicosis depends on the classification of the parasitosis. Localised cases can be kept under observation or receive a topical treatment with benzoyl peroxide to take advantage of its antiseborrhoeic qualities, which can create a more hostile environment for mites by eliminating the accumulation of sebum and keratin, which represent their sustenance. However, generalised cases should receive a more intense treatment.

Because secondary bacterial infections (especially those caused by *Staphylococcus pseudintermedius*) are very frequent and greatly complicate the clinical picture, consideration should be given to the possibility of treating patients with specific antibiotics (which often requires a bacterial culture and susceptibility testing) and topical antiseptics.

The patient received outpatient care. Glucocorticoids were discontinued and fluralaner was prescribed (1400 mg total every 3 months) plus oral cephalexin (30 mg/kg every 12 hours) and 2 baths per week with benzoyl peroxide. Treatment with fluralaner was initiated because of its safety and ease of administration. Cephalexin was used to treat the pyoderma given the presence of cocci in the cytological examination, and because the patient had not previously been prescribed oral antibiotics. Benzoyl peroxide has antimicrobial and keratolytic activity, which facilitates the exfoliation of hair follicles, thereby allowing the demodicosis and associated bacterial folliculitis to resolve.

Treatment alternatives

The treatment of choice for generalised cases of demodicosis was, for many years, amitraz at a concentration of 0.025 % in a bath every week or every 2 weeks. Although it is a drug that is not often used, it is still an option for the treatment of cases refractory to other more recent medications. Gloves, mask, goggles, and administration in a well-ventilated area are suggested for its application. To reduce the risk of poisoning, it is best to avoid applying it over the entire surface of the patient and to alternate administration on each side. After amitraz, ivermectin was the treatment of choice for demodicosis for a long time. Currently, it continues to be a good therapeutic option. The disadvantage of its use is that it requires the daily administration of a dose of 300–600 µg/kg body weight (in cats a dose of 300–500 µg/kg is suggested). For ivermectin to be effective, it must be administered daily. It is preferable to give it orally, since a daily injection can be painful for the patient. Usually, therapeutic doses are well tolerated, even for prolonged periods. Overdose may relatively rapidly cause signs of toxicity, such as mydriasis, vomiting, tremors, weakness and even seizures. Ivermectin-sensitive breeds (due to mutation in the ABCB1 gene, such as the Rough Collie, Border Collie, Bobtail, Australian Shepherd, Australian Cattle Dog, Shetland Shepherd, and Swiss White Shepherd) may show signs of toxicity at therapeutic doses. Other drugs related to ivermectin are currently still being used for the treatment of demodicosis. This is the case of other avermectins, such as doramectin (0.2–0.6 mg/kg), and milbemycins, such as moxidectin (0.2–0.5 mg/kg) and milbemycin oxime (0.5–2 mg/kg). Oral forms should be administered daily. Spot-on moxidectin may be given once weekly, while subcutaneous injectable doramectin may also be applied weekly. It should be noted that breeds susceptible to macrocyclic lactones may also be sensitive to therapeutic doses of doramectin, moxidectin or milbemycin oxime.

Currently, the most popular medication is fluralaner due mainly to two characteristics: it can be used very safely in breeds susceptible to ivermectin and it is administered every 3 months. Fluralaner belongs to the family of isoxazolines. This is a relatively recent family of gamma aminobutyric acid (GABA) and glutamate-dependent chloride channel blockers. Despite having a mechanism of action similar to macrocyclic lactones (such as ivermectin), it apparently binds to a site other than the receptor, in addition to the fact its (hepatic) metabolism takes a different path. The drug has low toxicity and has been shown to be effective against other external parasites, such as fleas, ticks and sarcoptes mites. It is not approved for use in cats.

CONCLUSION

At the next appointment, 1 month after beginning the treatment, the owners confirmed a marked improvement; Zeus's hair was beginning to regrow and his skin was not inflamed and did not have an unpleasant odour. The skin scrapings of the samples taken during the appointment showed the presence of 1–2 dead adult mites per area. The cytological examination was negative, so treatment with cephalexin was continued for 2 more weeks due to the presence of deep pyoderma at the initial appointment.

A skin scraping performed at the 2-month follow-up visit showed no evidence of the presence of parasites and the clinical signs had resolved (Fig. 6). Fluralaner was administered and the baths were continued, but their frequency was reduced (once a week) to avoid drying the skin.

At the 3-month follow-up visit, the owners were explained that the treatment must be continued for 1 month after obtaining 2 negative scrapings 1 month apart. Long-term monitoring was also discussed, with follow-up visits at 3 months, 6 months, and 1 year after the last negative scraping to ensure there was no relapse.

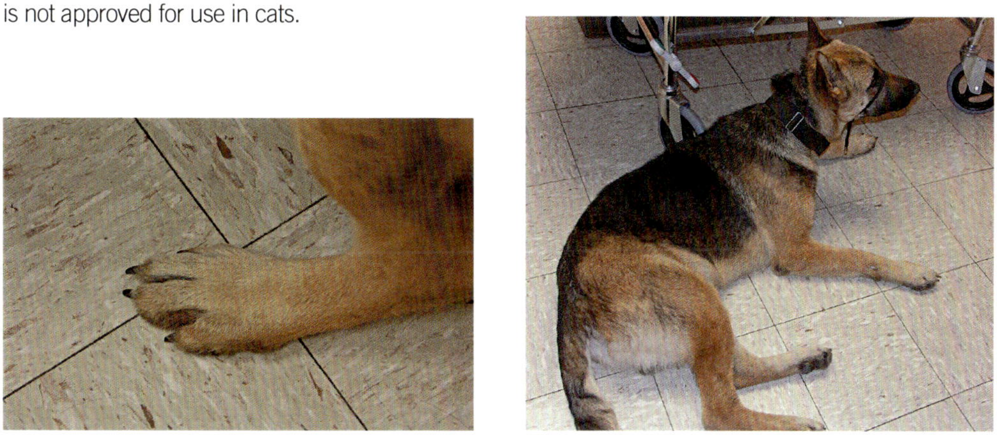

Figure 6. Resolution of the clinical signs after 2 months of treatment.

The prognosis of juvenile demodicosis is generally good, especially thanks to the availability of new effective treatments, which have a greater margin of safety. However, if there is an underlying, debilitating disease, demodicosis and secondary bacterial infections can turn into a complicated picture and produce serious sequelae, such as sepsis, thereby worsening the prognosis.

BIBLIOGRAPHY

Byrne KP. Metabolic epidermal necrosis-hepatocutaneous syndrome. *Vet Clin North Am Small Anim Pract.* 1999 Nov; 29(6): 1337–55.

Cosgrove SB, Wren JA, Cleaver DM *et al.* A blinded, randomized, placebo-controlled trial of the efficacy and safety of the Janus kinase inhibitor oclacitinib (Apoquel®) in client-owned dogs with atopic dermatitis. *Vet Dermatol.* 2013 Dec; 24(6): 587–97.

Ferrer Ll, Ravera I, Silbermayr K. Immunology and pathogenesis of canine demodicosis. *Vet Dermatol.* 2014 Oct; 25(5), 427–e65.

Fourie JJ, Liebenberg JE, Horak IG *et al.* Efficacy of orally administered fluralaner (Bravecto™) or topically applied imidacloprid/moxidectin (Advocate®) against generalized demodicosis in dogs. *Parasit Vectors.* 2015 Mar; 8: 187.

Griffin C. Otitis: anatomy every practitioner should know. *Compend Contin Educ Vet.* 2009 Nov; 31(11): 504–12.

Hall-Fonte DL, Center SA, McDonough SP *et al.* Hepatocutaneous Syndrome in Shih Tzus: 31 cases (1996–2014). *J Am Med Assoc.* 2016 Apr; 248(7): 802–13.

Ihrke PJ, Stannard AA, Ardans AA *et al.* Pemphigus foliaceus in dogs: a review of 37 cases. *J Am Vet Med Assoc.* 1985 Jan; 186(1): 59–66.

Miller W, Griffin C, Campbell K. Muller and Kirk's Small Animal Dermatology. Saunders 7th ed. 2012.

Mueller RS, Bensignor E, Ferrer Ll *et al.* Treatment of demodicosis in dogs: 2011 clinical practice guidelines. *Vet Dermatol.* 2012 Apr; 23(2), 86–e20.

Njaa B, Cole L, Tabacca, N. Practical Otic Anatomy and Physiology of the Dog and Cat. *Vet Clin North Am Small Anim Pract.* 2012 Nov; 42(6): 1109–1126.

Remedios AM, Fowler JD, Pharr JW. A comparison of radiographic versus surgical diagnosis of otitis media. JAAHA 1991; 27:183-188.

Rosenkrantz WS. Pemphigus: current therapy. *Vet Dermatol.* 2004 Apr; 15(2): 90–8.

Saridomichelakis MN, Olivry T. An update on the treatment of canine atopic dermatitis. *Vet J.* 2016 Jan; 207: 29–37.